# C APSICUM

## Therapeutic Powerhouse
## and Herbal Catalyst

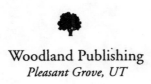

## Woodland Publishing
*Pleasant Grove, UT*

# CONTENTS

# INTRODUCTION

How many of us give the red hot chile pepper the respect it deserves? More often than not, most of us regard red pepper or Capsicum as nothing more than the spice added to give Cajun and Mexican cuisine its piquant kick. Technically speaking, cayenne pepper is the strongest red pepper variety of the *Capsicum* family, with paprika being the mildest.

Throughout this discussion, the terms *capsicum* and *cayenne pepper* will be used interchangeably. For our purposes, it's important to know that herbalists have designated both of these terms for the same botanical agent.

Health practitioners have known for centuries that Capsicum is much more than a culinary spice. Because they considered it a "hot" plant, Chinese physicians utilized it for physiologic conditions that needed stimulation. Capsicum or Cayenne Pepper is one of the few herbs that can be measured by its BTU or thermal units. In other words, it is a hot and stimulating pepper plant that can generate heat.

Recently, new and very valuable medicinal uses for Capsicum have emerged through scientific inquiry. The red chile pepper is experiencing a rediscovery among health care practitioners, who have only just begun to uncover its marvelous therapeutic actions. It has been referred to as the purest and most effective natural stimulating botanical in the herbal medicine chest.

The most recent clinical findings regarding Capsicum will be explored in our discussion with special emphasis on Capsicum's ability to heal ulcers, protect stomach mucosa and alleviate peripheral pain. Unquestionably, Capsicum exerts potent physiological and pharmacological effects without the side-effects commonly associated with powerful medicinal drugs.

Ironically, in the past, Capsicum's classification as a hot and spicy substance has done it a disservice. Because Capsicum is fiery and pungent, it is frequently regarded as dangerous and unpalatable. To the contrary, if it is used properly, Capsicum can be perfectly safe and impressively effective against a wide variety of physical disorders ranging from indigestion to ulcers to migraines. Its ability to lower blood cholesterol, boost circulation and even step up metabolism are worth serious consideration. In addition, its value for mental afflictions like depression must also be assessed. In a time when the notion of treating disease after the fact is more the rule than the exception, Capsicum offers protection from infectious invaders by boosting the effectiveness of the immune system. Today, amidst the over prescription of antibiotic drugs, Capsicum emerges as a potent immune fortifier, antioxidant and infection fighter.

A powerful compound called *capsaicin* is what gives Capsicum its bite and is also responsible for most of its beneficial effects on human physiology.[1] The hotter the pepper, the higher its content of capsaicin.[2] The remarkable properties of capsaicin will be discussed and documented clinical evidence supporting the use of capsaicin will be delineated.

It is important to realize in evaluating this herb that while it can be used alone, Capsicum is frequently added to herbal combinations to potentiate their overall action. This fact alone attests to the powerful but safe stimulant action of Capsicum. Stimulation is thought to be one of the keys to swift and complete healing.

Capsicum is ascending in prestige and is regarded as a modern-day botanical which is accruing new and impressive credentials. The fruit of this particular pepper plant is a valuable herbal treasure. It is vital to our health that we inform ourselves about its many medicinal uses.

# CAPSICUM (CAPSICUM ANNUUM)

*Common Names:* Cayenne Pepper, Red Pepper, African Bird Pepper, Bird Pepper, Spanish Pepper, American Red Pepper

*Plant Parts:* Fruit

*Active Compounds:* alkaloids (capsaicin), fatty acids, flavonoids, volatile oil, carotene pigment

*Nutritional Components:* Capsicum is rich in Vitamin C (ascorbic acid) and Zinc, two nutrients which are vital for a strong and healthy immune system. It is also high in vitamins, A, C, rutin (a bioflavonoid), beta carotene, iron, calcium and potassium. Capsicum also contains magnesium, phosphorus, sulphur, B-complex vitamins, sodium and selenium. The nutritional breakdown of Capsicum is as follows:

- Fats: 9-17%
- Proteins: 12-15%
- Vitamin A and red carotenoids (capsanthin, carotene, lutein)
- Ascorbic Acid (Vitamin C)
- B-Complex vitamins
- Potassium: 2014 mg per 100 edible grams
- Rutin (flavonoid)
- PABA

*Note:* Capsicum's red color is due in part to its very high content of vitamin A, which is vital for normal vision, cellular activity, growth and strong immune defenses.

*Pharmacology:* Capsaicin (active component) contains over 100 distinct volatile compounds.[3] It also contains capsacutin, capsaicin, capsantine, and capsico.

*Character:* analgesic, antibacterial, antioxidant, antipyretic, antiseptic, antispasmodic, aromatic, astringent, blood thinner, cardiovascular tonic, carminative, circulatory stimulant, diaphoretic, hemostatic, herbal accentuator, nerve stimulant, stomachic and tonic (general)

*Body Systems Targeted:* cardiovascular, circulatory, gastrointestinal, nervous, integumentary, skeletal, metabolic

*Herbal Forms:* loose dried powder, capsulized, tincture, infused oil, ointment or cream

*Usage:* Capsicum can be used liberally in a variety of forms. Capsulized dried Capsicum is probably the easiest and most practical way to take the herb. Commercial ointments can be purchased which contain from 0.025 to 0.075 percent capsaicin for the treatment of pain and psoriasis. Dried Capsicum can be mixed in hot water or can be used in tincture form, which can be added to water or juice.

*Safety:* Capsicum is generally recognized as safe in the United Sates and has been approved as an over-the-counter drug. A four week feeding study of Capsicum concluded, "It appears that red chile is relatively non-toxic at the doses tested in male mice."[4] The seeds of the fresh Capsicum plant should not be ingested. Doses of Capsicum should be followed precisely as prescribed to avoid gastrointestinal upset. Pregnant women or breast feeding mothers should avoid using Capsicum. Initial use of topical Capsicum can result in some skin irritation or burning; however, clinical tests have found that this diminishes with continued application. Avoid direct contact with eyes or other mucous membranes in general.

# HISTORY

Known to the natives of the tropical Americas for millennia, Capsicum, or Cayenne Pepper, was introduced to Europe by Christopher Columbus and became known as "Guinea Pepper." Originally used by Native Americans located south of the Mexican border, archeological evidence supports its cultivation from 7000 B.C. Apparently, mixing chocolate and red chiles was a taste treat exclusively reserved for Aztec royalty.[5]

The exact origin of the word *Capsicum* remains somewhat of a mystery. However, it is assumed to be a derivative of the Greek word *kapto*, meaning "to bite," an appropriate reference to its fiery pods. Capsicum is the fruit of a shrub-like tropical plant and is technically considered a berry. Its designation as a "pepper" can be traced back to Columbus, who equated its hot taste sensation with that of black pepper.

In 1597, Gerard referred to Capsicum as extremely hot and dry and prescribed it for throat and skin infections. Health practitioners of the nineteenth century called phsysiomedicalists used Capsicum to counteract rheumatism, arthritis, depression and chills. In the early 1800s, Dr. Samuel Thompson utilized Capsicum as a potent and safe natural stimulant. His followers, who would become known as Thomsonians, believed that Capsicum should be used to treat a wide variety of diseases. It was used orally and as a poultice to treat tumors, toothaches, fevers, and respiratory ailments.

In 1804, Dr. John Stevens introduced the red pepper to England where it became the catalyst component in a variety of herbal blends. Subsequently, herbal and medical practitioners used Capsicum to fight infection and sustain the natural heat of the body. It became well known in American dispensatories and pharmacopeia. In 1943, The Dispensary of the United States recorded that, "Capsicum is a powerful local stimulant, producing when swallowed, a sense of heat in the stomach and a general glow over the body without narcotic effect."[6]

Twentieth-century physicians recognized the medicinal value of Capsicum which eventually found its way to the *American Illustrated Medical Dictionary*, the *Merck Manual* and *Materia Medica,* where it was referred to as a rubefacient, local stimulant, counter-irritant, gastric stimulant, and diaphoretic.[7]

Today Mexican Indians continue to use Capsicum as an internal disinfectant and protectant against contaminated food and also to treat fevers.[8]

"Today the pepper is nowhere in the world more appreciated and more widely used than in Mexico and certain other Latin American countries, which together form the original home of all the peppers. Both at morning and at evening, practically every dish the Indians eat included Capsicum, just as their food did 2,000 years ago. The diet of the Indians was, and still is, rather bland . . . maize, beans, squash, pumpkin, yucca, potatoes . . . little wonder that the pepper was so highly regarded. And of course . . . the peppers were a wonderful source of essential vitamins in a diet otherwise lacking in them."[9]

Capsicum continues to be a source of vitality and health in numerous countries including the Bahamas and Costa Rica, where it is used to overcome colic or indigestion, in Africa for vascular disorders and by North Americans who use it as a tonic and natural stimulant.

Capsicum is currently experiencing a renaissance in that a number of recent studies have emerged adding to its already impressive list of actions. Scientists are taking notice and looking at Capsicum with new respect and interest. Perhaps what sets Capsicum apart is that unlike powerful pharmaceutical stimulants and pain killers, Capsicum possess potency without deleterious side effects.

# CLINICAL APPLICATIONS OF CAPSICUM

Capsicum is a remarkable whole body stimulant that can boost blood flow, tone the nervous system, relieve indigestion, promote sweating, help to cauterize and heal ulcers, ease persistent pain and fight off infection. One very authoritative work on African plants suggests that Capsicum's "regular ingestion is highly beneficial in hemorrhoids, varicose veins, anorexia, liver congestion and vascular conditions  . . .the indigenous inhabitants of Africa and of the Antilles are remarkably free form all of these conditions as they use Capsicum fruit in their diet."[10] Most of the therapeutic actions of Capsicum are attributed to the alkaloid or glucoside content of the herb.[11] The latest scientific studies conducted with Capsicum will be discussed in subsequent sections.

## Herbal Catalyst

Because Capsicum boosts peripheral circulation and stimulates organ secretion, it expedites the therapeutic delivery and action of other herbs. In other words, the medicinal benefits of these herbs reach infected or inflamed tissue more rapidly due to enhanced blood flow.[12] Consider the following statement:

"Cayenne will insure the rapid and even distribution of the active principles of the rest of the herbs to critical functional centers of the body, including those involved in cellular respiration, metabolism, data transmission, and neural-hormonal activation. Cayenne is included in several other blends for this reason. In extremely small quantities it can dramatically increase the efficiency of most other herbs."[13]

Many health practitioners believe that the key to healing is stimulation. Capsicum stimulates everything from blood flow to peristaltic action in the stomach, to intestinal transit time. The remarkable ability of Capsicum to stimulate organ secretion and even heart action makes it one of the strongest natural stimulants known. Several different kinds of herbal blends targeting various body systems will utilize Capsicum to boost the formula's efficacy.

# Cardiovascular Tonic

Capsicum is said to be unequaled for its ability to boost circulation and increase heart action. Interestingly, cultures who consume significant amounts of cayenne pepper in their diet have much lower rates of cardiovascular disease.[14] Capsicum exerts a variety of desirable actions on the entire cardiovascular system. It has the extraordinary ability to enhance cardiovascular performance while actually lowering blood pressure.[15]

A quote taken from a cardiovascular publication reads, "Capsaicin has also been shown to prolong cardiac action potential in atrial muscle . . ."[16] Michael T. Murray, N.D., has stated, "Cayenne pepper [Capsicum] should be recommended as a food for its beneficial antioxidant and cardiovascular effects."[17]

Herbalists have considered Capsicum as a superior "food" for the heart. In fact, in cases where a heart attack is suspected administering capsicum in hot water has been thought to help lessen the severity of the attack. Capsicum can also be placed on or under the tongue in emergencies involving heart attack, stroke or hemorrhaging.[18]

*Note:* Using Capsicum for any heart-related problem, especially a suspected heart attack should never take the place of medical attention or a physician's care.

# Blood Cholesterol Reducer

Various studies have conclusively demonstrated that Capsicum reduces the risk of developing atherosclerosis (hardening of the arteries) by reducing blood cholesterol and triglyceride levels.[19] Additional clinical studies conducted in India found that when cayenne was ingested along with dietary cholesterol, the typical rise in liver and blood serum cholesterol levels was significantly inhibited. In addition, bile acids and free cholesterol were subsequently eliminated from the body through the stool.[20]

Interestingly, these tests revealed that using Capsicum was actually more effective in reducing cholesterol that capsaicin alone.[21] Daniel Mowrey, Ph.D., emphatically points out that this is just one of many examples of the superiority of whole botanicals as opposed to their isolated components.[22]

*Note:* Using Capsicum in combination with Hawthorn is a particularly good cardiovascular tonic.

# Blood Pressure Equalizer

While an added bonus of Capsicum's capability to lower blood serum cholesterol is a decrease in blood pressure, additional evidence strongly suggests that the herb initiates other mechanisms that fight hypertension.[23] "Cayenne, according to another study, also reduces the blood pressure in an even more direct manner: a number of years ago, a team of researchers discovered that capsaicin acts in a reflexive manner to reduce systemic blood pressure, a kind of coronary chemoreflex."[24] Adding Garlic to Capsicum creates an even better therapeutic blend for treating hypertension.

# Blood Detoxification

"Cayenne is a kind of catalyst in the blood purification process . . . it acts as a diaphoretic, stimulating the excretion of wastes in the sweat."[25] Because Capsicum stimulates organ secretion and boosts peripheral blood flow, it would only stand to reason that it would also facilitate the faster removal of toxins from the bloodstream and lymphatic system. You may have already noticed that Capsicum is frequently added to blood-purifying herbal combinations.

# Circulatory Booster

Researchers have found that the simulating action of Capsicum on surface capillaries can help to prevent cold hands and feet.[26] For this reason, it may be helpful for Reynaud's Syndrome. Old remedies using Capsicum have even recommended placing it in socks to warm the feet and to help prevent frostbite. An old folk cure for a chilled body was a steaming hot cup of Capsicum tea.

# Free Radical Scavenger

The rich flavonoid content of Capsicum gives it significant antioxidant capabilities. A recent study conducted in 1995 showed that Capsicum has a higher ascorbic acid content than chiles from the jalapeno or serrano varieties.[27] Vitamin C and bioflavonoids can scavenge for dangerous free radicals which cause tissue damage and can predispose organs to degenerative diseases. Free radicals are found everywhere and are created as by-products of metabolic processes including the act of breathing itself. Pollutants can expose the body to free radicals. An interesting study done in Mexico City and published in 1993 found that Capsicum extract was able to modulate the mutagenic activity of urban air samples.[28] In other words, these potentially dangerous nitro-aromatic compounds found in polluted air were kept from mutating by red chile extract.[29] Chemical breakdowns of Capsicum have also found that the pepper is high in Provitamin A, which significantly contributes to its healing ability and immune fortification.[30]

# Anti-Carcinogenic Compound

Anti-cancer research recently tested Capsicum on laboratory rats and found that it does indeed demonstrate anti-cancer properties by inhibiting certain enzymes which can initiate the mutation of cells.[31] What this implies is that taking Capsicum can afford the body some protection against the cellular mutation which occurs in malignant growths. Capsicum actually inhibited the formation of dangerous metabolites under laboratory conditions where they should have normally been activated.[32] This study implies that Capsicum may have many more sophisticated bio-chemical actions than previously thought.

# An Impressive Pain Killer

Capsaicin has recently emerged as a remarkably effective pain reliever and has become the subject of recent clinical research. Applying capsaicin in cream or ointment form to painful joints, scar tissue or other painful conditions involving peripheral nerves confuses pain transmitters. In other worlds, capsaicin temporarily disrupts sensory nerve cell biochemistry thereby impeding the relay of pain sensations from the skin surface. It does this by inhibiting a neurotransmitter called substance P. This specific compound is thought to be the main mediator of pain impulses from peripheral nerve endings.[33] Substance P has also demonstrated its ability to inhibit inflammatory pain generated in arthritic joints in much the same way.[34]

Today, several over-the-counter topical preparations utilize capsaicin for the pain of arthritic joints. The ability of Capsicum to control severe and unresponsive pain is significant, to say the least. Modern clinical utilization of topical capsaicin may offer significant relief for a number of painful conditions including: diabetic neuropathy, cluster headaches, post-amputation pain, post-mastectomy pain, shingles and painful scar tissue.[35]

## POST-SURGICAL PAIN

In the early spring of 1996, prime time national news shows reported that scientists had found that individuals who had suffered from chronic pain in post-surgical scars (heart bypass, arterial grafts, etc.) were successfully treated with topical preparations containing capsaicin. While this may have been news to many of us, clinical studies had been already published for several years that capsaicin held profound value for various kinds of pain which did not respond to established medical treatments. Typically surgical scars and regions around them can produce persistent pain or can be very sensitive to the touch even when completely healed. This type of pain phenomenon seems to respond well to capsaicin ointments and creams.

## POST-MASTECTOMY PAIN

When capsaicin preparations were applied following mastectomy or breast reconstruction, pain was significantly relieved. Several double blind studies found that using capsaicin creams four times daily for 4 to 6 weeks resulted in much less frequent occurrence of sharp, jabbing pain.[36] All thirteen patients studied had a 50 percent or greater improvement.[37] Various unpleasant sensations other than pain also improved with topical applications of capsaicin creams.[38]

## MOUTH SORES FROM RADIATION OR CHEMOTHERAPY

A fascinating study conducted at the Yale Pain Management Center discovered that capsaicin could very significantly lessen pain caused by mouth sores which frequently develop after chemotherapy or radiation.[39] Apparently delivering the capsaicin in the form of soft candy (taffy) enabled the substance to be retained in the mouth long enough to desensitize the nerve endings causing the pain. Each one of the eleven case studies reported that their pain had decreased and in two patients, it stopped entirely.[40]

## DIABETIC NEUROPATHY

Diabetic neuropathy is a painful nerve condition which can develop in cases of prolonged diabetes. Several double-blind studies have supported the considerable value of capsaicin creams for relieving the pain associated with this disorder.[41]

The results of a controlled study using Capsicum for severe cases of diabetic neuropathy which did not respond to conventional therapy were published in 1992. A cream containing Capsicum was applied to painful areas four time a day and pain was carefully evaluated for 8 weeks at two-week intervals. The results were impressive, to say the least. In the 22 patients who used the Capsicum the following results were recorded: "Capsaicin treatment was more beneficial than vehicle treatment in the overall clinical improvement of pain status, as measured by physician's global evaluation and by a categorical pain severity scale . . . In a follow-up study, approximately 50 percent of the subjects reported improved pain control or were cured . . ."[42]

*Note:* While there was a burning sensation when the Capsicum cream was first applied, some subjects found that its magnitude and duration lessened with continued application.[43]

## SHINGLES

The FDA has approved capsaicin-based ointments for the treatment of pain that results from diseases like shingles. Again, numerous studies have documented the value of capsaicin for decreasing the miserable nerve-related pain associated with shingles. The general consensus derived from these tests were that approximately 50 percent of people suffering from shingles responded well to cap-saicin creams, some even after 10 to 12 months.[44]

*Note:* If blisters accompany a shingles outbreak, it is better to wait until they have healed before using any capsaicin-based ointments or creams.

## RELIEF FOR BURNING FEET

Frequently an uncomfortable "burning" sensation in the feet will occur in many people, particularly in diabetics. As ironic as it may seem, using capsaicin creams may actually alleviate this burn-ing. "In various studies, diabetics who treated their burning feet with capsaicin got greater improvement and were able to walk more easily than those not using the cream."[45] In addition, using topical applications of capsaicin as opposed to strong, oral drugs is much more preferable.

## ARTHRITIS PAIN

Clinical tests have confirmed that topical capsaicin ointments substantially alleviate the miserable pain that characterizes osteo- and rheumatoid arthritis.[46] These studies revealed that using 0.075 capsaicin cream reduced tenderness and pain.[47]

Dr. Michael T. Murray writes:

" . . . seventy patients with osteoarthritis and thirty-one with rheumatoid arthritis received capsaicin or placebo for 4 weeks. The patients were instructed to apply 0.025 per-cent capsaicin cream or its placebo to painful knees four times daily. Significantly more relief of pain was reported by the capsaicin-treated patients than by the placebo patients throughout the study . . ."[48]

Anyone suffering from osteo or rheumatoid arthritis should evaluate the effectiveness of capsaicin ointments for joint pain.

Ester Lipstein-Kresch, M.D., has studied the effectiveness of capsaicin creams for arthritis and has stated: "You need to apply it three or four times a day on the affected area for at least two weeks before you'll see any improvement. An initial burning sensation at the site is not unusual for the first few days, but this goes away with continued application."[49]

*Note:* Capsaicin is also useful for tennis elbow due to its ability to block the transmission of pain.

## MIGRAINE HEADACHES (CLUSTER TYPE)

Topical applications of capsaicin ointments intranasally may also help to relieve the pain of a specific kind of migraine headache called cluster headaches. Cluster headaches are characterized by severe pain which typically radiates around one eye. The term "cluster" refers to the fact that these headaches tend to occur in clusters of one to three per day and can recur at  intervals. Headache pain and severity were reducing in groups using intranasal capsaicin.[50] This type of capsaicin treatment should be done under a physician's care. There is some speculation that capsaicin may be more effective in preventing migraines before they develop into a full blown attack.[51]

# Stomach Ulcers

Ironically, if you suffer from a peptic or duodenal ulcer, the last thing you feel probably feel inclined to take is hot Cayenne Pepper. While it goes against everything we've ever heard about what aggravates an ulcer, the facts are that most "spicy" foods do just the opposite. Capsicum has the ability to serve as a local anesthetic to ulcerated tissue and can even help to control bleeding.

While some individuals may be bothered by eating "peppery" or spicy foods, these foods do not cause the formation of gastric ulcers in normal people. What is particularly interesting is that people suffering from ulcers who would normally avoid Cayenne Pepper, may actually benefit from its therapeutic action.

In addition, taking Capsicum may significantly reduce the risk of ever developing a peptic ulcer. A Chinese study published in 1995 stated, "Our data supports the hypothesis that the chile used has a protective effect against peptic ulcer disease."[52]

Another 1995 study found that Capsicum can even protect the stomach lining from aspirin induced ulcers.[53] As most of us are aware, aspirin can cause stomach ulceration in certain individuals if a sensitivity exists or if taken with too little liquid. Researchers concluded after experiments with human volunteers that the capsaicin content of capsicum has a pronounced gastro-protective effect on the mucous membranes of the stomach.[54] Eighteen healthy volunteers with normal gastrointestinal mucosa took chile and water followed by 600 mg of aspirin and water. The study was conducted over a period of four weeks. Endoscopy results showed that taking 20 gm of chile before the aspirin definitely demonstrated a protective action on the stomach lining.[55] In short, Capsicum has the ability to rebuild stomach tissue.

*Note:* The ability of Capsicum to bring blood to regions of tissue at a faster rate boosts the assimilation of foods that are consumed with it.[56] Several clinical studies support this phenomenon. It is thought that Capsicum initiates the release of certain substances which increase secretions and facilitate better profusion of blood to the stomach and intestines.[57] Capsicum can increases the flow of digestive secretions from the salivary, gastric and intestinal glands.

# Capsicum and the Gastro-Intestinal Tract

In 1992, researchers tested the effect of chile or Capsicum on gastrointestinal emptying. Eight healthy volunteers were evaluated before and after the addition of Capsicum to their meals. The results conclusively demonstrated that the ingestion of Capsicum greatly effects intestinal transit time.[58] If food moves faster through from the stomach through the intestines, caloric assimilation and bowel evacuation may be influenced for the better. Capsicum seems to "speed up" various physiological processes. To add transit time to the list of functions Capsicum boosts comes as somewhat of a surprise and additional benefit.

## Capsicum and Weight Loss

Capsicum may be an unheralded weight loss aid that is perfectly safe to use. Studies have suggested that Capsicum can slow fat absorption in the small intestines and actually boost the metabolic rate so the thermogenesis (fat burning) is enhanced.[59] In many instances excessive weight gain is thought to be a result of a sluggish metabolism. Capsicum has been singled out by herbalists as an herb which may boost the burning of fat.[60] Unlike other stimulants, Capsicum does not cause palpitations, hyperactivity or a rise in blood pressure. For this reason, it may be a valuable weight loss supplement that has been generally overlooked.

## Psoriasis

As mentioned earlier, capsaicin has the ability to inhibit a neurotransmitter called substance P. Interestingly, an excess of substance P has been associated with psoriasis. Michael T. Murray, in his book, *The Healing Power of Herbs,* points out that this finding led researchers to study the effects of capsaicin ointments on psoriasis.[61] Regarding the use of such an ointment for psoriasis, he states:

" . . . In one double-blind study, forty-four patients with symmetrically distributed psoriasis lesions applied topical capsaicin to one side of their body and a placebo to the other side. After 3 to 6 weeks, significantly greater reductions in scaling and redness were observed on the capsaicin-treated side. Burning, stinging, itching, and skin redness were noted by nearly half of the patients initially, but these diminished or vanished on continued applications."[62]

There is no question that capsaicin based ointments should be employed for psoriasis. Tests have conclusively found that treating psoriasis with capsaicin caused significant improvement in a variety of symptoms as well as the severity of the attack.[63]

# Rhinitis

Capsicum has also scientifically proven its value in people suffering from vasomotor rhinitis. By using Capsicum in spray form, researchers found that it was able to significantly reduce nasal obstruction and secretion.[64] It is important to understand that in these particular instances, a Capsicum solution was applied directly to the mucous membranes of the nose. It did initially cause a painful burning and stimulated nasal secretion. However, in time, after repeated applications, these side effects disappeared.[65] Apparently, Capsicum may block the action of peripheral nerve endings which may stimulate nasal secretion and blockage. More study of Capsicum as a viable treatment for rhinitis has been recommended.

*Note:* One of the many properties of Capsicum is its ability to break up mucous congestion which makes expectoration much easier.[66] For this reason, Capsicum is recommended for upper respiratory infections which are characterized by excess mucus.

# Fever and Chills

While it may seem somewhat contradictory, Capsicum actually lowers the temperature of the body by stimulating the region of the hypothalamus, which cools the body.[67] "The ingestion of cayenne peppers by cultures native to the tropics appears to help these people deal with high temperatures."[68] Capsicum also promotes perspiration which helps to cool the body off. In tropical areas, local people eat substantial amounts of hot peppers on a daily basis which helps to boost the elimination of sweat and thereby keeps body temperature down.

This same mechanism can be used to treat fever and chills. In addition to this action, using Capsicum for any infection that may be causing a fever is also warranted. Capsicum helps to boost immune defenses and fights microorganism invasion.

# Capsicum, Infection and Immune Power

Capsicum not only stimulates organ secretion and circulation, it has a tonic effect on the immune system, making the body less vulnerable to microorganism invaders. Dr. John R. Christopher writes of an artist who observed that natives of Coyoacan, Mexico seemed to be particularly resistant to intestinal infection. He writes:

"He [the artist] observed that the natives had a remarkable immunity to amoebic dysentery due to their fondness of raw chile peppers which they ingested in tremendous quantities as part of their normal diet."[69]

In addition to intestinal infections, Capsicum has significant value for upper respiratory ailments including colds, influenza, sore throats etc. Because it can increase blood flow to peripheral tissues, it insures the better deliver and assimilation of nutrients which are required by infected areas in order to heal quickly. This same action enhances the removal of waste material and toxins from inflamed areas thereby facilitating faster recovery. Whatever area of the body is afflicted, it is imperative that blood supply is adequately infused over the region. The constituents of the immune system which include macrophages, T-cells, etc., are blood-borne, therefore the better capillary delivery of blood, the faster the healing process can occur.

A study published in 1994 found that Capsicum even had the ability to exert an anti-giardia effect in vitro.[70] The effect of Capsicum was so impressive that a notation was made that its performance was considered superior to tinidazol (the pharmaceutical drug used to treat Giardia).[71]

## The Preventive Power of Capsicum

Taking daily doses of Capsicum can help to protect the body from colds, flu, sore throats, other bacterial or viral infections, heart disease, indigestion and fatigue.[72] Capsicum is frequently combined with Garlic to create a potent immune system fortifier.

## Capsicum for Fatigue and Depression

The natural stimulatory action of capsicum can provide better performance under conditions of stress. Laboratory studies involving animals which were stressed under a variety of conditions, performed better if Capsicum was added to their diet the day before testing.[73] In addition, this study discovered that Capsicum was not as effective if taken two to three days prior to evaluation, indicating that its results were short-lived.[74]

Other studies found that the ability of Capsicum to stimulate circulation and respiratory reflexes may help to enhance physiologic performance under periods of stress or fatigue.[75] Scientists in France have accrued additional evidence that taking Capsicum does indeed help to counteract fatigue.[76]

In addition to physical stress, mental disorders like depression may also respond to the stimulating effect of Capsicum. Many health practitioners look upon depression as a "slowing down" of brain impulses and neurochemical reactions. Because Capsicum can increase peripheral blood flow and promote cellular function, its usage for mental disorders like depression should be further evaluated. Traditionally, pungent aromatics like clove have been utilized through aroma therapy to uplift the spirits and invigorate the mind. Capsicum works much in the same way.

"Cayenne or Capsicum helps to stimulate circulation and has an energizing effect on the system. It has traditionally been used for overcoming fatigue and restoring stamina and vigor. It is considers a natural stimulant without the side effects of most stimulating agents."[77]

# SUMMARY OF SPECIFIC ACTIONS ASSOCIATED WITH CAPSICUM

The following are specific actions associated with capsicum and the conditions it can help relieve.

- can help to stop both internal and external hemorrhaging
- facilitates the healing of ulcers
- high flavonoid content makes it a good antioxidant
- boosts heart action without raising blood pressure
- improves the ratio of HDL to LDL cholesterol
- supports vessel and capillary elasticity
- helps to protect against heart disease and stroke
- may help to minimize damage from heart attack or shock
- works to re-build and heal injured stomach tissue
- rich in vitamin C, it strengthens the immune system
- promotes better digestion by boosting HCL secretion
- acts to equalize blood pressure
- may help to increase thermogenesis or the burning of fat
- topical use relieves pain of arthritis, surgical scars, shingles etc.
- used on the skin, may help to protect against frostbite

- serves as a powerful catalyst for other herbs
- helps to relieve psoriasis

# PRIMARY MEDICINAL APPLICATIONS OF CAPSICUM

appetite stimulant

arthritis

asthma

atherosclerosis

bleeding (internal and external)

blood pressure

bronchitis

burning feet

chills

circulatory disorders

colds

congestion

depression

diabetic neuropathy

fatigue

frostbite (prevention)

heart ailments

heart attack

hemorrhage

indigestion

infection

laryngitis

migraines (cluster headaches)

mouth pain

nausea

nosebleeds

general pain

phlebitis

pleurisy

psoriasis

rheumatism

shock

sore throat

strokes

tennis elbow

tonsillitis

toothache

ulcers

varicose veins

wound bleeding

## Substances that Complement Capsicum

As previously mentioned, Capsicum is frequently added to herbal combinations in order to boost and potentiate their action. The following herbs create particularly good herbal complements with Capsicum: garlic, ginger, hawthorn berry, peppermint, myrrh, yucca, gotu kola, parsley, rosemary, echinacea, kelp, ginseng, ginkgo, bayberry, slippery elm, black walnut, papaya, peppermint, fennel, St. John's Wort, and lobelia.

# CONCLUSION

The fiery hot red chile pepper arrived in our hemisphere in the 16th century. It has only been recently, since science has begun to validate Capsicum's medicinal use, that the herb has gained the prestige it deserves. Capsicum is one of the most potent whole-body stimulants with a whole array of therapeutic actions. Ironically, while many of us are turning to antacids, antibiotics and over-the-counter pain relievers, Capsicum may offer us the most curative benefits with the least side effects. You can be certain that when it comes to using Capsicum for health related conditions, we have only seen the tip of the iceberg. Clearly, Capsicum should be utilized more fully as a medicinal staple. It should be considered nothing less than a wonder herb that has scientifically proven its worth. What Mexican and African natives have known for centuries could most definitely enhance our health and well-being.

# ENDNOTES

1 G.A. Cordell and O.E. Araujo, "Capsaicin: Identification, nomenclature, and pharmacotherapy." *Ann. Pharmacother.* 27: 1993, 330-336.
2 A.Y. Leung. *Encyclopedia of Common Natural Ingredients used in Food.* (John Wiley and Sons, New York: 1980.
3 Cordell, 330-36.
4 J.J. Jang, D.E. Defor, D.L. Logsdon and J.M. Ward. "A 4-week feeding study of ground red chile (Capsicum annuum) in male mice." *Food-Chem-Toxicol.* Sept. 1992 30 (9): 783-7.
5 John R. Christopher. *Capsicum.* (Christopher Publications, Springville, Utah: 1980), 27.
6 Jack Ritchason. *The Little Herb Encyclopedia,* 3rd ed. (Woodland Publishing, Pleasant Grove, Utah: 1994), 44.
7 Christopher, 4.
8 Juliette Bairacli-Levy. *Common Herbs for Natural Health.* (Schocken Books, New York: 1974), 41-43.
9 Charles B. Heiser. *Nightshades.* (W.H. Freeman, San Francisco: 1969), 18.
10 Lenden H. Smith, M.D., E.P. Donatelle, M.D., Vaughn Bryant, Ph.D. et al. *Basic Natural Nutrition.* (Woodland Books, Pleasant Grove, Utah: 1984), 157.
11 J. Jurenitsch et al. "Identification of cultivated taxa of Capsicum: taxonomy, anatomy and composition of pungent principle." *Chemical Abstracts.* 91 July 30, 1977: 35677g.
12 Daniel B. Mowrey. *The Scientific Validation of Herbal Medicine.* (Keats Publishing, New Canaan, Connecticut: 1986), 159.
13 Ibid., 208-09.
14 Michael T. Murray. *The Healing Power of Herbs, 2nd ed.* (Prima Publishing, Prima, California: 1995), 71.
15 J. De Lille and E. Ramirez. "Pharmacodynamic action of the active principles of chile (capsicum annuum L.) *Anales Inst. Biol.* 1935: 6, 23-37. See also C.C. Toh, T.S. Lee et al. "The pharmacological actions of capsaicin and its analogues." *British Journal of Pharmacology.* 1955: 10, 175-182.
16 N.A. Castle. "Differential inhibition of potassium currents in rat ventricular myocytes by capsaicin." *Cardiovasc-Res.* Nov. 1992, 26 (11): 1137-44.
17 Murray, *The Healing Power of Herbs,* 72.
18 Ritchason, 46.
19 T. Kawada, et al. "Effects of capsaicin on lipid metabolism in rates fed a high fat diet." *Journal of Nutrition.* 1986: 116, 1272-78. See also J.P. Wang, et al. "Antiplatelet effect of capsaicin." *Thrombosis Res.* 1984: 36, 497-507, and S. Visudhiphan, et al. "The relationship between high fibrinolytic activity and daily capsicum ingestion in Thais." *American Journal of Clinical Nutrition.* 1982: 35, 1452-58.
20 K. Sambaiah and N. Satyanarayana. "Hpocholesterolemic effect of red pepper and capsaicin." *Indian Journal of Experimental Biology.* 1980: 18, 898-99. See also M.R. Srinivasan, et al. "Influence of red pepper and capsaicin on growth, blood con-

stituents and nitrogen balance in rats." *Nutrition Reports International.* 1980: 21 (3): 455-67.

21 Mowrey, 12.

22 Ibid.

23 Toh, 175-182.

24 Mowrey, 12.

25 Ibid., 19-20.

26 Louise Tenney. *The Encyclopedia of Natural Remedies.* (Woodland Publishing, Pleasant Grove, Utah: 1995), 42. See also Peter Holmes. *The Energetics of Western Herbs.* (Artemis Press, Boulder: 1989), 322.

27 Y. Lee, et al. "Flavonoids and antioxidant activity of fresh pepper (Capsicum annuum) cultivars." *Journal of Food Science.* May 1995: 60 (3): 473-76. See also L.R. Howard, et al. "Provitamin A and ascorbic acid content of fresh pepper cultivars (Capsicum annuum) and processed jalapenos." *Journal of Food Science.* March, 1994: 59 (2): 362-65.

28 J.J. Espinosa-Aguirre, et al. "Mutagenic activity of urban air samples and its modulation by chile extracts." *Mutat-Res.* Oct. 1993: 303 (2): 55-61.

29 Ibid.

30 Howard, 362-65.

31 Z. Zhang, S.M. Hamilton, et al. "Inhibition of liver microsomal cytochrome P450 activity and metabolism of the tobacco-specific nitrosamine NNK by capsaicin and ellagic acid." *Anticancer-Res.* Nov-Dec. 1993: 13 (6A): 2341-46.

32 C.H. Miller, Z. Zhang, et al. "Effects of capsaicin on liver microsomal metabolism of the tobacco-specific nitrosamine NNK." *Cancer-Lett.* Nov. 30, 1993: 75 (1): 45-52.

33 Murray, *The Healing Power of Herbs,* 71.

34 Cordell, 330-36. See also Murray, *The Healing Power of Herbs,* 70-71.

35 Murray, *The Healing Power of Herbs,* 72.

36 C.P.N. Watson, et al. "The post-mastectomy pain syndrome and the effect of topical capsaicin." Pain. 1989: 38, 177-86. See also C.P.N. Watson and R.J. Evans. "The post-mastectomy pain syndrome and topical capsaicin: A randomized trial." *Pain.* 1992: 51, 375-79.

37 Murray, *The Healing Power of Herbs,* 73.

38 Watson, 177-86.

39 C. Nelson. "Heal the burn: Pepper and lasers in cancer pain therapy." *Journal of the National Cancer Institute.* 1994: 86, 1381.

40 Ibid.

41 "The capsaicin study group: Effect of treatment with capsaicin on daily activities of patients with painful diabetic neuropathy." *Diabetes Care.* 1992: 15, 159-65. See also R. Tanden, et al. "Topical capsaicin in painful diabetic neuropathy. Effect on sensory function." *Diabetes Care.* 1992: 15, 8-14, K.M. Basha and F.W. Whitehouse. "Capsaicin: A therapeutic option for painful diabetic neuropathy." *Henry Ford Hospital Medical Journal.* 1991: 39, 138-40, and M.A. Pfeifer, et al. "A highly successful and novel model for treatment of chronic painful diabetic peripheral neuropathy." *Diabetes Care.* 1993: 16, 1103-15.

42 R. Tanden, et al. "Topical capsaicin in painful diabetic neuropathy: controlled study with long- term follow-up." *Diabetes Care.* Jan. 1992: 15 (1): 8-14.

30 ✳ CAPSICUM

43 Ibid.
44 J.E. Bernstein, et al. "Topical capsaicin treatment of chronic post-herpetic neuralgia (shingles) with topical capsaicin. A preliminary study. *Journal of American Academy of Dermatologists.* 1987: 17, 93-96. See also Murray, The Healing Power of Herbs, 72.
45 Sid Kircheimer. *The Doctor's Book of Home Remedies.* (Rodale Press, Emmaus, Pennsylvania: 1993), 228.
46 Murray, *The Healing Power of Herbs,* 74.
47 G.M. McCarthy and D.J. McCarty. "Effect of topical capsaicin in therapy of painful osteoarthritis of the hands." *Journal Rheumatol.* 1992: 19, 604-07. See also C. L Deal, et al. "Treatment of arthritis with topical capsaicin: A double blind trial." *Clinical Therapy.* 1991: 13, 383-95.
48 Murray, *The Healing Power of Herbs,* 74.
49 Kircheimer, 14.
50 Murray, *The Healing Power of Herbs,* 74.
51 Michael T. Murray, N.D. and Joseph Pizzorno, N.D. *Encyclopedia of Natural Medicine.* (Prima Publishing, Rocklin, California: 1991), 419.
52 J. Y. Kang, et al. "The effect of chile ingestion of gastrointestinal mucosal proliferation and azoxymethane-induced cancer in the rat." *Journal of Gastroenterology-Hepatol.* Mar-Apr. 1992: 7 (2): 194-98.
53 K. G. Yeoh, et al. "Chile protects against aspirin-induced gastroduodenal mucosal injury in humans." *Dig-Dis-Sci. Mar.* 1995: 40 (3): 580-83.
54 Ibid.
55 Ibid.
56 L. Limlomwongse, et al. "Effect of capsaicin on gastric acid secretion and mucosal blood flow in the rat." *Journal of Nutrition.* 1979: 109, 773-77. See also T. Kolatat and D. Chungcharcon. "The effect of capsaicin on smooth muscle and blood flow of the stomach and the intestine." *Siriraj Hospital Gazette.* 1972: 24, 1405-18, O. Ketusinh, et al. "Influence of capsaicin solution on gastric acidities." *American Journal of Proceedings.* 1966: 17, 511-15, and Mowrey, 48.
57 Mowrey, 48 and Limlomwongse, 773-77.
58 M. Horowitz, et al. "The effect of chile on gastrointestinal transit." *Journal of Gastroenterology-Hepatol.* Jan-Feb, 1992 7 (1): 52-56.:
59 Christopher Hobbs. "Cayenne, This Popular Herb is Hot." *Let's Live.* April 1994: 55.
60 V. Badmaev and M. Majeed. "Weight loss, the Ayurvedic system." *Total Health.* Aug, 1995: 17 (4): 32-35.
61 Murray, *The Healing Power of Herbs,* 75.
62 C.N. Ellis, et al. "A double-blind evaluation of topical capsaicin in pruritic psoriasis." *Journal of the American Academy of Dermatology.* 1993: 29 (3): 438-42.
63 Murray, *The Healing Power of Herbs,* 75.
64 S. Marabini, et al. "Beneficial effect of intranasal applications of capsaicin in patients with vasomotor rhinitis." *Eur Arch-Otorhinolaryngol.* 1991: 248 (4): 191-94.
65 Ibid.
66 Mowrey, 242.
67 B. Dib. "Effects of intrathecal capsaicin on autonomic and behavioral heat loss responses in the rat. *Pharmacol Biochem Behav.* 1987: 28, 65-70.
68 Murray, *The Healing Power of Herbs,* 72.

69 Christopher, 31.
70 M. Ponce, et al. " In vitro effect against giardia of 14 plant extracts." *Rev-Invest-Clin.* Sept- Oct. 1994: 46 (5): 343-47.
71 Ibid.
72 Humbart Santillo. *Natural Healing with Herbs.* (Hohm Press, Prescott, Arizona: 1993), 100.
73 Daniel B. Mowrey. "Capsicum ginseng and gotu kola in combination." *The Herbalist* premier issue, 1975: 22-28.
74 Ibid.
75 Mowrey, *The Scientific Validation of Herbal Medicine,* 102.
76 J. Roquebert, et al. "Study of vasculotropic properties of Capsicum annuum." *Annales Pharmaceutiques Francaises.* 1978: 36 (7-8): 361-68.
77 Rita Elkins. *Depression and Natural Medicine.* (Woodland Publishing, Pleasant Grove, Utah: 1995), 161.